100 Races
A Running Journal

Dr. Emily Schwartz

This journal belongs to:_____

DISCLAIMER

This journal is not meant to be medical advice. Always consult a doctor before beginning an exercise program. Please don't push yourself. It could take you 5 years to fill out this journal. It could take you 50. It's ok!

"Running is nothing more than a series of arguments between the part of your brain that wants to stop and the part that wants to keep going."-Unknown

AUTHOR'S NOTE

My running journey began on Amazon.com at 2:00AM. I was never really an athlete. I was more of the "let's stand motionless against the wall and hope the teacher doesn't see us" type of student in P.E. As I got older, I had a million excuses for why I didn't exercise. "Grad school keeps me too busy" then "kids keep me too busy" then "it's too hot," "my legs hurt," "gyms are expensive." I had uttered them all.

Then, one evening, something just snapped. I was sick of excuses. I was sick of telling myself I "wasn't athletic." As I sat, wide awake, looking at the running shoes in my Amazon cart wondering if spending this $50 would be enough to make me stick to an exercise plan for more than a few weeks, I had no idea what type of journey I was about to embark on.

Fast forward a year, and I'm about to celebrate my 1 year "runniversary." I went from hardly being able to run for 60 seconds, to completing four 5Ks and two 4 milers. I'm currently training for two 10Ks and I couldn't be happier with what running has done for my life. I'm healthier. I'm in the best shape of my life. I'm setting a great example for my children. I no longer have to awkwardly avoid eye contact when my doctor asks how often I exercise.

But I realized that without a goal, I ran the risk (pun intended) of my running journey becoming stale. I needed a big goal. A HUGE one. A goal so big it didn't seem feasible. That's how I settled on "100 Races" and I want YOU to join me.

Love,
Emily

How to Use This Book
It doesn't matter if you complete this book over the course of several years or a lifetime. It doesn't matter if you fill it with 5Ks or full marathons. The purpose of this book is to see how far you've come and track your progress as you experience your own running journey.

Recording Your Stats
For each race, record the date, name, location, distance, time, and average pace. The "other" line is reserved for any other data you are interested in tracking. For example, you might want to track your heart rate, your weight, your water intake, your pre-race meal, etc.

Memorable Moments
This is where you include anything fun or different about the race. Try to be specific! It's fun to look back on your running memories. For example, did you run the race with a friend? Was it your first time sporting some new running shoes? Was it extra hot? Extra cold? Be sure to record any little details that will help you remember the race later.

How to Improve
You'll also have the opportunity after each race to reflect on how to improve for next time. One of the greatest rewards of self reflection is the opportunity for self growth. How can you use your race experience to get better next time? You may want to make notes about how much water to drink, what foods to eat, great play lists to use, or what time to arrive at the race. We always assume we'll remember these lessons that experience teaches us, but we won't unless we write them down.

Finally, have fun! I'm so glad to be on this running journey with you.

How did you start your running journey?

Race #1   Date:

Race Name:

Location:

Distance:

Time:

Pace:

Other:

Memorable moments:

How to improve next time:

Race #2

Date:

Race Name:

Location:

Distance:

Time:

Pace:

Other:

Memorable moments:

How to improve next time:

Race #3   Date:

Race Name:

Location:

Distance:

Time:

Pace:

Other:

Memorable moments:

How to improve next time:

Race #4

Date:

Race Name:

Location:

Distance:

Time:

Pace:

Other:

Memorable moments:

How to improve next time:

Race #5   Date:

Race Name:

Location:

Distance:

Time:

Pace:

Other:

Memorable moments:

How to improve next time:

Race #6

Date:

Race Name:

Location:

Distance:

Time:

Pace:

Other:

Memorable moments:

How to improve next time:

Race #7

Date:

Race Name:

Location:

Distance:

Time:

Pace:

Other:

Memorable moments:

How to improve next time:

Race #8   Date:

Race Name:

Location:

Distance:

Time:

Pace:

Other:

Memorable moments:

How to improve next time:

Race #9   Date:

Race Name:

Location:

Distance:

Time:

Pace:

Other:

Memorable moments:

How to improve next time:

Race #10

Date:

Race Name:

Location:

Distance:

Time:

Pace:

Other:

Memorable moments:

How to improve next time:

Race #11

Date:

Race Name:

Location:

Distance:

Time:

Pace:

Other:

Memorable moments:

How to improve next time:

Race #12   Date:

Race Name:

Location:

Distance:

Time:

Pace:

Other:

Memorable moments:

How to improve next time:

Race #13

Date:

Race Name:

Location:

Distance:

Time:

Pace:

Other:

Memorable moments:

How to improve next time:

Race #14   Date:

Race Name:

Location:

Distance:

Time:

Pace:

Other:

Memorable moments:

How to improve next time:

Race #15

Date:

Race Name:

Location:

Distance:

Time:

Pace:

Other:

Memorable moments:

How to improve next time:

Race #16

Date:

Race Name:

Location:

Distance:

Time:

Pace:

Other:

Memorable moments:

How to improve next time:

Race #17   Date:

Race Name:

Location:

Distance:

Time:

Pace:

Other:

Memorable moments:

How to improve next time:

Race #18

Date:

Race Name:

Location:

Distance:

Time:

Pace:

Other:

Memorable moments:

How to improve next time:

Race #19

Date:

Race Name:

Location:

Distance:

Time:

Pace:

Other:

Memorable moments:

How to improve next time:

Race #20

Date:

Race Name:

Location:

Distance:

Time:

Pace:

Other:

Memorable moments:

How to improve next time:

Race #21

Date:

Race Name:

Location:

Distance:

Time:

Pace:

Other:

Memorable moments:

How to improve next time:

Race #22

Date:

Race Name:

Location:

Distance:

Time:

Pace:

Other:

Memorable moments:

How to improve next time:

Race #23

Date:

Race Name:

Location:

Distance:

Time:

Pace:

Other:

Memorable moments:

How to improve next time:

Race #24

Date:

Race Name:

Location:

Distance:

Time:

Pace:

Other:

Memorable moments:

How to improve next time:

Race #25   Date:

Race Name:

Location:

Distance:

Time:

Pace:

Other:

Memorable moments:

How to improve next time:

Race #26

Date:

Race Name:

Location:

Distance:

Time:

Pace:

Other:

Memorable moments:

How to improve next time:

Race #27

Date:

Race Name:

Location:

Distance:

Time:

Pace:

Other:

Memorable moments:

How to improve next time:

Race #28

Date:

Race Name:

Location:

Distance:

Time:

Pace:

Other:

Memorable moments:

How to improve next time:

Race #29

Date:

Race Name:

Location:

Distance:

Time:

Pace:

Other:

Memorable moments:

How to improve next time:

Race #30　　Date:

Race Name:

Location:

Distance:

Time:

Pace:

Other:

Memorable moments:

How to improve next time:

Race #31

Date:

Race Name:

Location:

Distance:

Time:

Pace:

Other:

Memorable moments:

How to improve next time:

Race #32

Date:

Race Name:

Location:

Distance:

Time:

Pace:

Other:

Memorable moments:

How to improve next time:

Race #33

Date:

Race Name:

Location:

Distance:

Time:

Pace:

Other:

Memorable moments:

How to improve next time:

Race #34   Date:

Race Name:

Location:

Distance:

Time:

Pace:

Other:

Memorable moments:

How to improve next time:

Race #35

Date:

Race Name:

Location:

Distance:

Time:

Pace:

Other:

Memorable moments:

How to improve next time:

Race #36

Date:

Race Name:

Location:

Distance:

Time:

Pace:

Other:

Memorable moments:

How to improve next time:

Race #37

Date:

Race Name:

Location:

Distance:

Time:

Pace:

Other:

Memorable moments:

How to improve next time:

Race #38   Date:

Race Name:

Location:

Distance:

Time:

Pace:

Other:

Memorable moments:

How to improve next time:

Race #39   Date:

Race Name:

Location:

Distance:

Time:

Pace:

Other:

Memorable moments:

How to improve next time:

Race #40

Date:

Race Name:

Location:

Distance:

Time:

Pace:

Other:

Memorable moments:

How to improve next time:

Race #41

Date:

Race Name:

Location:

Distance:

Time:

Pace:

Other:

Memorable moments:

How to improve next time:

Race #42

Date:

Race Name:

Location:

Distance:

Time:

Pace:

Other:

Memorable moments:

How to improve next time:

Race #43

Date:

Race Name:

Location:

Distance:

Time:

Pace:

Other:

Memorable moments:

How to improve next time:

Race #44

Date:

Race Name:

Location:

Distance:

Time:

Pace:

Other:

Memorable moments:

How to improve next time:

Race #45   Date:

Race Name:

Location:

Distance:

Time:

Pace:

Other:

Memorable moments:

How to improve next time:

Race #46

Date:

Race Name:

Location:

Distance:

Time:

Pace:

Other:

Memorable moments:

How to improve next time:

Race #47

Date:

Race Name:

Location:

Distance:

Time:

Pace:

Other:

Memorable moments:

How to improve next time:

Race #48   Date:

Race Name:

Location:

Distance:

Time:

Pace:

Other:

Memorable moments:

How to improve next time:

Race #49   Date:

Race Name:

Location:

Distance:

Time:

Pace:

Other:

Memorable moments:

How to improve next time:

Race #50

Date:

Race Name:

Location:

Distance:

Time:

Pace:

Other:

Memorable moments:

How to improve next time:

Race #51

Date:

Race Name:

Location:

Distance:

Time:

Pace:

Other:

Memorable moments:

How to improve next time:

Race #52   Date:

Race Name:

Location:

Distance:

Time:

Pace:

Other:

Memorable moments:

How to improve next time:

Race #53

Date:

Race Name:

Location:

Distance:

Time:

Pace:

Other:

Memorable moments:

How to improve next time:

Race #54

Date:

Race Name:

Location:

Distance:

Time:

Pace:

Other:

Memorable moments:

How to improve next time:

Race #55

Date:

Race Name:

Location:

Distance:

Time:

Pace:

Other:

Memorable moments:

How to improve next time:

Race #56

Date:

Race Name:

Location:

Distance:

Time:

Pace:

Other:

Memorable moments:

How to improve next time:

Race #57

Date:

Race Name:

Location:

Distance:

Time:

Pace:

Other:

Memorable moments:

How to improve next time:

Race #58

Date:

Race Name:

Location:

Distance:

Time:

Pace:

Other:

Memorable moments:

How to improve next time:

Race #59   Date:

Race Name:

Location:

Distance:

Time:

Pace:

Other:

Memorable moments:

How to improve next time:

Race #60

Date:

Race Name:

Location:

Distance:

Time:

Pace:

Other:

Memorable moments:

How to improve next time:

Race #61

Date:

Race Name:

Location:

Distance:

Time:

Pace:

Other:

Memorable moments:

How to improve next time:

Race #62

Date:

Race Name:

Location:

Distance:

Time:

Pace:

Other:

Memorable moments:

How to improve next time:

Race #63   Date:

Race Name:

Location:

Distance:

Time:

Pace:

Other:

Memorable moments:

How to improve next time:

Race #64   Date:

Race Name:

Location:

Distance:

Time:

Pace:

Other:

Memorable moments:

How to improve next time:

Race #65

Date:

Race Name:

Location:

Distance:

Time:

Pace:

Other:

Memorable moments:

How to improve next time:

Race #66   Date:

Race Name:

Location:

Distance:

Time:

Pace:

Other:

Memorable moments:

How to improve next time:

Race #67

Date:

Race Name:

Location:

Distance:

Time:

Pace:

Other:

Memorable moments:

How to improve next time:

Race #68

Date:

Race Name:

Location:

Distance:

Time:

Pace:

Other:

Memorable moments:

How to improve next time:

Race #69

Date:

Race Name:

Location:

Distance:

Time:

Pace:

Other:

Memorable moments:

How to improve next time:

Race #70

Date:

Race Name:

Location:

Distance:

Time:

Pace:

Other:

Memorable moments:

How to improve next time:

Race #71   Date:

Race Name:

Location:

Distance:

Time:

Pace:

Other:

Memorable moments:

How to improve next time:

Race #72

Date:

Race Name:

Location:

Distance:

Time:

Pace:

Other:

Memorable moments:

How to improve next time:

Race #73

Date:

Race Name:

Location:

Distance:

Time:

Pace:

Other:

Memorable moments:

How to improve next time:

Race #74

Date:

Race Name:

Location:

Distance:

Time:

Pace:

Other:

Memorable moments:

How to improve next time:

Race #75

Date:

Race Name:

Location:

Distance:

Time:

Pace:

Other:

Memorable moments:

How to improve next time:

Race #76

Date:

Race Name:

Location:

Distance:

Time:

Pace:

Other:

Memorable moments:

How to improve next time:

Race #77

Date:

Race Name:

Location:

Distance:

Time:

Pace:

Other:

Memorable moments:

How to improve next time:

Race #78

Date:

Race Name:

Location:

Distance:

Time:

Pace:

Other:

Memorable moments:

How to improve next time:

Race #79   Date:

Race Name:

Location:

Distance:

Time:

Pace:

Other:

Memorable moments:

How to improve next time:

Race #80

Date:

Race Name:

Location:

Distance:

Time:

Pace:

Other:

Memorable moments:

How to improve next time:

Race #81

Date:

Race Name:

Location:

Distance:

Time:

Pace:

Other:

Memorable moments:

How to improve next time:

Race #82

Date:

Race Name:

Location:

Distance:

Time:

Pace:

Other:

Memorable moments:

How to improve next time:

Race #83

Date:

Race Name:

Location:

Distance:

Time:

Pace:

Other:

Memorable moments:

How to improve next time:

Race #84

Date:

Race Name:

Location:

Distance:

Time:

Pace:

Other:

Memorable moments:

How to improve next time:

Race #85   Date:

Race Name:

Location:

Distance:

Time:

Pace:

Other:

Memorable moments:

How to improve next time:

Race #86　　　Date:

Race Name:

Location:

Distance:

Time:

Pace:

Other:

Memorable moments:

How to improve next time:

Race #87

Date:

Race Name:

Location:

Distance:

Time:

Pace:

Other:

Memorable moments:

How to improve next time:

Race #88

Date:

Race Name:

Location:

Distance:

Time:

Pace:

Other:

Memorable moments:

How to improve next time:

Race #89

Date:

Race Name:

Location:

Distance:

Time:

Pace:

Other:

Memorable moments:

How to improve next time:

Race #90

Date:

Race Name:

Location:

Distance:

Time:

Pace:

Other:

Memorable moments:

How to improve next time:

Race #91   Date:

Race Name:

Location:

Distance:

Time:

Pace:

Other:

Memorable moments:

How to improve next time:

Race #92

Date:

Race Name:

Location:

Distance:

Time:

Pace:

Other:

Memorable moments:

How to improve next time:

Race #93

Date:

Race Name:

Location:

Distance:

Time:

Pace:

Other:

Memorable moments:

How to improve next time:

Race #94   Date:

Race Name:

Location:

Distance:

Time:

Pace:

Other:

Memorable moments:

How to improve next time:

Race #95

Date:

Race Name:

Location:

Distance:

Time:

Pace:

Other:

Memorable moments:

How to improve next time:

Race #96

Date:

Race Name:

Location:

Distance:

Time:

Pace:

Other:

Memorable moments:

How to improve next time:

Race #97

Date:

Race Name:

Location:

Distance:

Time:

Pace:

Other:

Memorable moments:

How to improve next time:

Race #98   Date:

Race Name:

Location:

Distance:

Time:

Pace:

Other:

Memorable moments:

How to improve next time:

Race #99　　Date:

Race Name:

Location:

Distance:

Time:

Pace:

Other:

Memorable moments:

How to improve next time:

Race #100   Date:

Race Name:

Location:

Distance:

Time:

Pace:

Other:

Memorable moments:

How to improve next time:

100 Races

YAY!
Congratulations!! You did it!! Did you ever think you could do it?? Now what ELSE sounds impossible? What else sounds too difficult to accomplish? Go DO it because you CAN and you're AMAZING!

Love, Emily

100 Races

www.ingramcontent.com/pod-product-compliance
Lightning Source LLC
Chambersburg PA
CBHW081657270326
41933CB00017B/3203